I0787464

Foreword

Welcome,

In advance, I would like to thank some people who have supported me through this case study.

First of all, I would like to thank the Healthcare Team from the sheltered living organization for the support throughout this training. They have made it possible for me to grow during training as a human and Mental Health Care Worker.

My practical counsellor, Linda, has always assisted me with advice and assistance to complete this Guide and case study.

Also the people of the pharmacy on the domain of the Psychiatric Center have assisted me with advice, and provided with literature.

Finally, I would like to thank Bie for guiding my project as well as Mimi for the professional support in the field and in the sessions Supervision.

Enjoy reading

[Type here]

TOC

'The Health Group' is the name of practical implementation in this Guide and case study.

This initiative aims to develop an efficient way that is applicable and adaptable at all times, in accordance with a specific group of sheltered living participants with a view to promoting a healthy lifestyle.

The focus is on integrating healthy, balanced and varied diets and not on losing weight. No measurements of the[1] participants' abdominal circumference, fat percentage, weight or BMI are deliberately taken.

The health group wants to inform, raise awareness, support and teach skills in a process of changing their own eating and exercise behavior.

This Guide and case study contains 8 chapters to make the learning process and realization transparent.

In the first chapter you will learn more about our provision and vision outlined as well as the infrastructure classification.

---

[1] Body Mass Index

My own history and personal vision are described in this chapter as this is a starting point of my motivation and passion for this subject.

The second chapter describes the stated objectives of this Guide and case study. These objectives are arranged chronologically and are distinguished in the short, medium and long term.

Chapter three deals with the question, the complexity and the influencing factors on the problem within our setting.

Gaining a better understanding of the issue is central.

Here we focus on our team's experiences in practice, as well as the interaction between psychological, physical and social vulnerability of the target group and participants.

The fourth chapter highlights theoretical and scientific frameworks that are used as tools to tackle the problem as efficiently as possible. Here we take a broad look at all possible influences at both the micro level and the macro level.

They relate to everyone in society and therefore also to people of sheltered living.

Chapter 5 explains the exploration of the various interventions such as ambivalence as a point of contact and the use of algorithms.

Chapter 6 shows the Guide for the various information sessions. The approach to achieving the objectives is set out in this chapter.

The preparation and the course of the information sessions can be found in chapter 7. Both the content, agenda items and the group dynamics are explained.

Chapter 8 explains the effects of the health group on the participants.

It provides advice for further guidance.

The objectives achieved and not achieved are clarified and justified, as well as the future prospects of the health group.

1. DESCRIPTION OF CONTEXT AND PERSONAL JUSTIFICATION

1.1 PRACTICAL PRESENTATION AND TARGET GROUP

In the finalisation phase of this integrated test, I was employed for about 1 year in this organisation.

Before, I did two years of internship within the same organisation of sheltered living. Most people come after a long stay in a psychiatric centre to this place. See it as a period between to hospitalisation and life in society.

We have 50 approved places for people with long-term psychiatric problems and a psychosocial issue. This makes us visible in the region.

Our target group consists of a heterogeneous, vertical group of adults.

Next primary diagnoses on AS-I from DSM-IV for our residents (Annual Report, 2015)

Ψ   14 people have a psychotic disorder, mainly of the
Ψ   schizophrenic type
Ψ
Ψ   9 people with mood disorder, mainly recurrent
Ψ   depression and bipolar disorder
Ψ
   2 persons with an amnestic disorder due to alcohol

   5 people with a behavioral disorder

   4 people with anxiety disorder

   3 people with amnestic disorder such as impulse
      disorder/somatization disorder/dissociative disorder

Ψ   3 people without diagnosis
Ψ
   5 persons with substance dependence other than
   alcohol

This initiative for sheltered living, 10 group houses are present with an offer of different housing options.

We have 6 community houses, 3 residential properties that allow living in a studio for 14 residents and 1 studio which is suitable for a couple to live together.

Each supervisor takes care of an integral approach to the individual resident... This results in a varied set of tasks such as ADL guidance, budget guidance, administrative support, follow-up medication intake, ... In addition to individual guidance, guidance from a group of residents is also part of the tasks.

We provide an average of 3 counselling
moments per week for each resident.

The vision of the guidance focuses on the optimal
development of the capacities of each resident and the
realization of a normal and meaningful existence for
each resident. We focus on reintegrating our residents
into society and encouraging the preservation and/or
restoration of social contacts (family, friends, social)

Chronically ill individuals need emotional support and
improve the quality of their lives. [2] The theme of my
thesis fits in with this last point. The physical condition of
a person undoubtedly has a direct influence on the
quality of life.

1.2 PROFILE OF THE PARTICIPANTS[3]

Caroline

Psychological diagnosis: Psychosis

Physical diagnosis: Breast cancer (cured)

Caroline is a severely psychotic woman who now
functions relatively stable. Stable is the first
impression she gives but there are still positive[4]
schizophrenic symptoms present. These are 5
votes that affect her thinking.

These voices are her friends.

She enjoys the moments to sit in the seat in her
studio listening to her voices. This withdrawal
behavior is covered by the negative[5] symptoms
of schizophrenia. She is gentle and pleasant in
dealing but her extreme obesity and the strain of
her pathology mortgage her energy levels to get
through the day.

She takes 5 different types of antipsychotics and two
types of benzodiazepines.[2] Despite this sedating and
heavy medication, she is at most times alert and
talkative.

Marieke

Psychological diagnosis: Alcohol dependence

Marieke is a 60-year-old woman. She's had a lot to drink
throughout her life. As a result of this lifestyle it has
mildly demented symptoms such as confusion and
orientation problems.

For her, loneliness and depression lurk around
the corner. In order to activate the activities, the

---

[2] Benzodiazepines have a specific effect on anxiety and can be used as a
sedative. They can highly excited patients. Benzodiazepines can amplify
the problems associated with addiction and induce additional addiction.

(Psychopharmacology Manual, 2012)

guidance must always be intensively present. Cognitively it functions at a low level.

Anneke

Psychological diagnosis: Psychosis

Anneke is a woman with average intelligence who comes from a family where psychosis is strongly present.

2   People talk about 'optimal' quality of life for people in outpatient care if one starts to function positively in the following areas of life: personal development, self-determination, interpersonal relationships, social inclusion, rights, emotional well-beingphysical well-being, material well-being. (Boevinck, Wolf, C, & A, 1995)

3   In this final work, fictitious names are of course used for the participants to guarantee the privacy of the client. 4 Positive means not "good" here, but that there is something that someone didn't have before.

5 Negative is mentioned in psychosis if someone loses things that he/she previously had,

She is verbally strong and knows what she wants in life. Her fear of blemishing, which is reinforced by a psychotic train of thought, before that, living with others has not been a success.

This is why she's staying at a studio. Things are much better here, she is very independent, manages all ADL tasks, can manage her correspondence herself and she ensures that there is always sense of day care.

From an early age and from my pre-education Physical Education and Sport (A2) I have always had an interest in movement and everything that has to do with it.

Those who exercise of uses energy and reserves that the body possesses.

In order to exercise daily, it is therefore essential to have the right knowledge and to have the right eating habits, so that one can supplement the reserves that the body has.

In this way, over the years my interest in exercise and nutrition has grown.

Maintaining a healthy lifestyle is a challenge for most of us.

My personal motivation is also socially focused when one knows that 80 percent of strokes are a result of heart disease and type 2 diabetes and 40 percent of cancer cases could be avoided if one were to change people's lifestyles. (European Commission, 2007) During this Orth pedagogics course I took the time to do about 6 weeks of volunteer working a shelter for homeless children in Nairobi, Kenya, during the summer of 2013. The first 5 days of my stay in Nairobi I participated in a CHE[3] training. This was given by American missionaries with the intention of making a change in the community of health education. It addressed very mundane health problems that were scientifically correct and substantiated. This course brought a good translation to individuals and communities from remote regions where the level of education often does not exceed primary school level.

In these regions, there are often many different theories and explanations to fight and cure certain diseases based on faith and experience, but which are usually not scientifically based.

This training trained us to work with the CHE handbook to provide health education through this route with the aim: raising awareness of the community.

I was able to test this training in practice by teaching the children at the shelter. Both the experiences of this trip and the experiences of other destinations I have undertaken to developing countries have given me more shape as a person and made me think about our standard of living and the consequences of it.

---

[3] Community Health Evangelism.

Once back in my own country, after every trip, I was robbed with an oversupply of products and brands during the first visit to the supermarket.

At the beginning of the 20th century it was mainly shortages that led to all-out diseases in our country.

But in today's society, most attention is focused on health problems caused by overconsumption.

The economic boom of the 1960s and 1970s increased our standard of living.

Due to our high standard of living and cunning marketing techniques, the oversupply of food products and the demand for them was increasing.

In most cases, oversupply leads to overnutrition[4]. This results in overweight and overweight related diseases. Here we are talking about the average Belgian. But add to this fact that we are dealing here with people with mental disorders. These individuals often have a greater lack of exercise than the average Belgian because of the direct consequences (e.g. depression) or indirect consequences (e.g. medication use) of their disorder.

---

[4] 'Overnutrition' means we have a greater absorption of energy and macronutrients (proteins, fats and carbohydrates) than the body burns due to the basic metabolism (at rest) and psychological and physical exertion.

All this plays into my conviction and motivation to work around nutrition and exercise.

<hr>

2. OBJECTIVES

❖ Goal A: Inform and raise awareness: Participants are made aware of what a healthy lifestyle means

The participants are present and show their cooperation at the weekly information sessions for six weeks. The participant question their own behavior and attitude in a critical way and become aware of their own lifestyle and its consequences.

❖ Purpose B: To promote eating and exercise: There are visible changes in the daily life of the participant

The handles and insights they are given to promote eating and exercise during the information sessions and individual moments are applied in daily life.

❖ Goal C: Changes and objectives have been implemented in the client's guidance plan

In order to guarantee the continuity of the objectives and to maintain the change process of the participants, the findings, observations and experiences have been included in the individual guidance plans.

- ❖ Goal D: The Guide for the health group has been drawn up

The Guide contains an overview of all direct preparatory activities, power point slides, attachments, nutrition tests as well as an overview of the necessary material for each session.

All information about the target, the health problem, the goal to be achieved are comprehensively defined in this Guide and case study that serves as a supported part of the Guide .

The already appointed successor of the health group takes this playbook over. This bundling is delivered at the completion of this project.

3. INFLUENCING FACTORS OF THE ISSUE

3.1 INTERACTION BETWEEN PSYCHOLOGICAL, PHYSICAL AND SOCIAL VULNERABILITY

During the counselling moments, we, as an accompanying family, are often amazed at the eating habits of our residents.

More logically, the guidance always points to this unhealthy behavior, but there is still no initiative within our setting that will focus specifically on this problem.

The idea has been around for several years to work more deeply on the eating and movement behavior of our people.

Besides my personal motivation, there is also a great motivation and encouragement from the team to follow this up in practice.

There are initiatives towards physical activity. For example, the residents are encouraged and motivated to participate in the joint walk every Friday afternoon. When we speak of a successful turnout, it can be said that 1 in 4 residents participated in this walking afternoon.

ANOTHER REGULAR HEARING FOR THE ATHLETES IS ON THURSDAY AFTERNOON. AT THAT TIME, A RECOGNIZED SPORTS ORGANIZATION FOR PEOPLE WITH MENTAL HEALTH PROBLEMS ORGANIZES A SPORTS AFTERNOON IN THE URBAN SPORTS HALL. THE TURNOUT IS DETERMINED IN 1 IN 4 RESIDENTS. FOR THIS, WE TRY TO MOTIVATE OUR

Increased appetite, drowsiness, lethargy, passivity,
sedation, are just some of the many possible side effects
of psychiatry medication.

These make the step towards exercise and healthy eating
seem much greater than for those without psychiatric
medication.

Unfortunately, some people living in sheltered shelters
who take antipsychotics are clearly affected by these
side effects.

Patients taking antipsychotic are at risk of numerous
physical side effects.[5] When one speaks of weight gain,
one will have to look at the first time if one can change
something about the diet and lifestyle changes.
It is known that changes in eating and lifestyle have only
a slight impact on body weight. Here the body weight will
stagnate rather than be reduced and this only with a very
disciplined diet.

It is clozapine and Olanzapine in particular that greatly
increase the risk of weight gain.

---

[5] See Annex 1 for a detailed diagram ofthe usual antipsychotic medication
and their consequences.

The person in treatment may have already gained 20 kilos after the first two months.

This will continue to increase if no steps around diet and lifestyle are taken.

Change of the drug is not an option if one knows that these products are often the last resort.

This weight gain in turn increases the risk of Metabolic syndrome[6] that will cause complications other than the direct effects, of antipsychotics use. (Cahn, et al., 2008) In addition, one also has the general psychological vulnerability, which negatively affects eating and exercise behavior.

Research (Psychiatric function disorders in vulnerable elderly people, 2010) has shown that people with many psychological complaints, such as depressive feelings, have a higher risk of physical illness, including poor self-care, malnutrition, reduced mobility, social isolation and emotional capacity. Eating, smoking and using alcohol or drugs are bad habits that some people have to deal with stress.

Patients with schizophrenia smoke more often and more than the average citizen.

---

[6] Metabolic syndrome is a combination of 3 out of 5 following somatic abnormalities: increased glucose – and triglyceride value, reduced concentration of high-density lipoprotein cholesterol, tintra-abdominal fatty tissue and hypertension.

Quitting smoking can even lead to epileptic on-all, in patients taking Clozapine.

(Psychopharmacology Manual, 2012).

In other words, there seems to be a strong interaction between psychological, physical and social vulnerability.

If one has to take long-term heavy psychiatric medication, which is accompanied by little physical activity, one will be predatory on one's own body over the years.

Limited gift ability that leads to ignorance when choosing the right products in the supermarket is another important factor.

People with limited talent are very susceptible to the many marketing strategies that supermarkets apply.

These individuals are guided by the easiest and most obvious choice.

After all, many residents are wrongly convinced that they eat and cook healthily. When I take stock of these poor eating habits in combination with a lack of physical activity, there is a clear imbalance.

However, it is possible to overcome all these obstacles and opt for a healthy lifestyle in terms of nutrition and exercise.

That's why I saw the need to work with some people of sheltered living, taking into account and becoming

vigilant for their psychological vulnerability, needs and
needs.

3.2 A SOCIAL PHENOMENON

As you can see from the following graph (Figure 1),
derived from a large-scale examination of the health
survey (Bayingana, Demarest, & Gisle, 2004), the gap in
health status between the low and the highly educated is
widening.

This is a social phenomenon that is clearly also
manifesting itself within sheltered living. Within our
setting, the percentage of low-skilled workers[7], at the
time of this thesis (census took place in January 2015), is
65.38%.

---

[7] They are considered to be low-skilled if they do not obtain a diploma or
certificate of secondary education. People from part-time vocational
secondary education are also considered to be low-skilled Considered.
(VDAB, 2010)

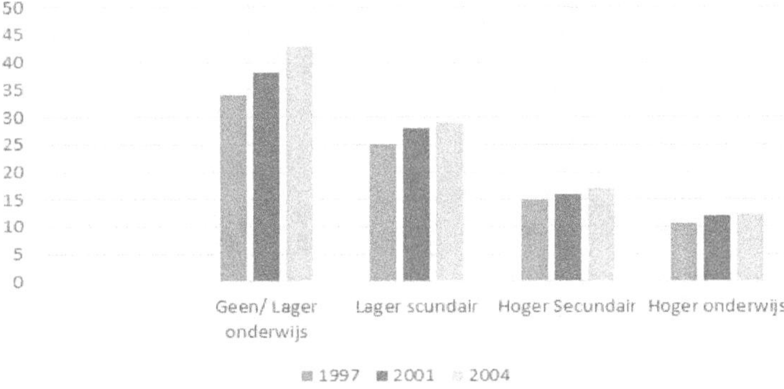

FIGURE 1 - Gap in health status between
low and high-skilled

In terms of the most educated, less educated people are relatively more likely to smoke, exercise less, have an unhealthier diet and are also less likely to change that pattern.

(Buziarsist & Gisle, 2001)

However, this problem perpetuates itself when one knows that 'deprivation leads to poor health and poor health leads to deprivation ' (Buziarsist & Gisle, 2001) It is precisely this group of lower-skilled people where, in our daily guidance, we have a clear need and demand for support in this.

Another causal fact of the problem is the lack of proper knowledge.

This of course goes hand in hand with the above described part.

This ignorance entails the wrong choice when purchasing products in the supermarket.

3.3 SEDENTARY BEHAVIOR

Sedentary behavior refers to activities in which energy consumption does not far exceed resting metabolism.

Activities that fall under sedentary behavior include: sitting, lying, WATCHING TV and other forms of 'screen-based entertainment'.

During counselling moments I see the sedentary behavior in all shapes, sizes and positions. For adults, it is very important to minimize sedentary behavior. In periods of inactivity, they lose more muscle mass and strength than young people.

Research has shown that after one day of rest, middle-aged people need about two weeks of physical activity to regain the same level of muscle strength than before bed rest (Beers, Jones, & Berkwits, 2008).

4. THEORETICAL FLOOR

4.1 STAGES OF BEHAVIORAL CHANGE (PROCHASKA, NORCROSS, & DICLEMENTE, 1994)

4.1.1 INTRODUCTION

The model of the stages of behavioral change, is a model that is often used in addiction care. In order to get out of the downward spiral, more logical behavioral change is needed.

This change in behavior can only be successful if one sees the negative consequences of the behavior and one has alternatives to address the real problems.

Prochaska and Diclemente proved in 1994 from research that behavioral change often seems to be via a fixed pattern. (Prochaska, Norcross, & Diclemente, 1994) They found a model with 5 consecutive stages.

As can be seen in Figure 3 (Van Der Veen & Goijarts, 2008), there are change processes at every stage that we, as supervisors, have to respond to. It is therefore crucial that these phases can be identified before they can be intervened. In practice, the stages do not seem to be as strongly bounded. The time perspective on which they follow each other can also fluctuate very much.

During 1 conversation or 1 counselling moment, the person in question can move from one stage to the next and vice versa.

This model is useful in detecting the ambivalence[8] of the client. It is precisely here that we have to intervene to start the process of change.

It is important to go further into these conflicting feelings. This is what we call exploring ambivalence. As a counsellor, you help the resident to explore his ambivalence by engaging in conversation and letting the patient articulate what he thinks is rich.   A tool for this is to create a balance. This means that you explore and name all the pros and cons of unhealthy life.

It is important to have an eye for both sides of the balance. This reduces the chance of resistance and creates space to think about change. The resident feels understood and experiences that the conversation is about what is essential to him, not about what should be.

———————————————————

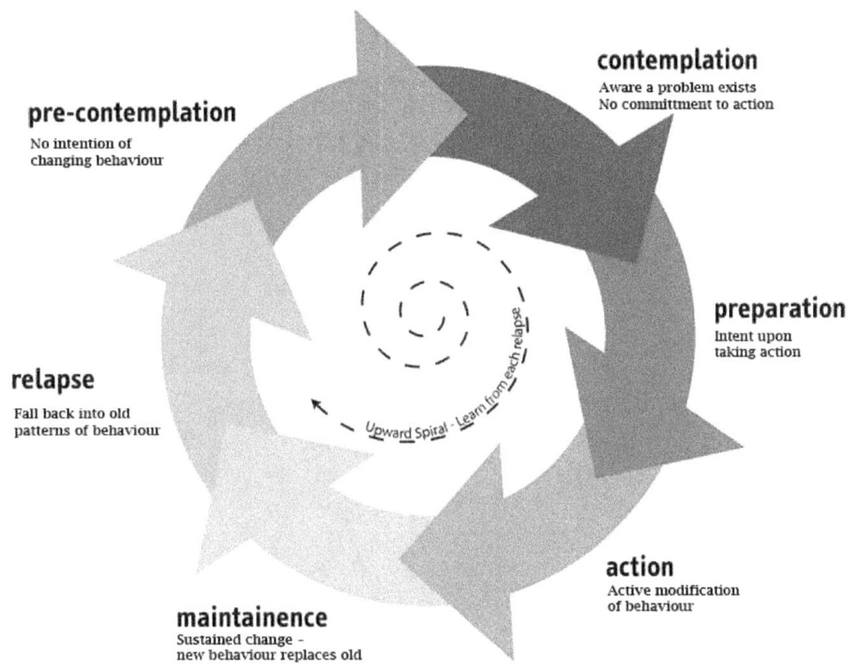

FIGURE 3 – Phases of behavioral change

4.1.2 THE FIRST PHASE: PRE-PHASE OR PRECONTEMPLATION

Denial and reasoning away from the problem are very characteristic here.

Here people have no intention of changing their behavior
in the near future. Two groups of people are found here.

- Unconsciously: those who are not aware of the
  problem or the risk they run. *Possible thinking: ' I
  eat enough vegetables, why should I eat more? "*

- Conscious: Those who know that there is a
  problem but oppose it.

  *Possible thinking: ' I go to the bus every day on
  foot, about 5 minutes walk. That's enough
  exercise, isn't it? My GP recommends something
  different to me, but I feel good about this
  choice.'*

4.1.3 THE SECOND PHASE: CONTEMPLATION OR CONTEMPLATION PHASE

At this stage, people are aware of a problem. We have
already thought about changing, but no concrete plans
are being made. There is a danger here that one will
remain stuck at this stage. Here there are conflicting or
ambivalent feelings present. This phase sometimes
becomes the 'Yes, but...' phase.

*Possible thinking: ' I should lose weight, but... I might be
able to take a walk.*

4.1.4 THE THIRD PHASE: PLANNING OR PREPARATION PHASE

What is very characteristic of this phase is that they are thinking about what they want to change. Information and help are being sought to make this happen.

There may be some barriers to being overcome or skills being taught here.

Behavior has not changed at this stage.

Possible thinking: 'I will start changing within two weeks. Get a fitness subscription next week. The day after tomorrow my diet will start.""

4.1.5 THE FOURTH PHASE: THE PHASE OF ACTION

Here one is only started (up to 6 months) in changing his or her behavior. The behavior is effectively adapted to the goal that comes first.

Often this adjustment is made in steps.

A resident said: 'I used to eat nothing fruit and now I eat one piece a day.'

At this stage, achievable and realistic objectives must be set once a goal has been achieved. The ultimate goal is to achieve a healthy lifestyle.

To achieve this, an adjustment of the environment and behavior is required.

The well-behaved behavior is often not continuous and there will be ups and downs. *Possible thinking: ' I always go to work by bike, unless it rains.'*

At this stage, there is an assertive person present, which teaches them to maintain their behavior and skills. It is said that conservation is carried out over a period of time between 6 months and 5years.

Possible thinking: 'These changes are part of my daily schedules. I'm not white bread anymore now that I've switched to brown bread. If I didn't walk, I miss it, too.

Here there is no longer any tendency to set back the old behavior. The new behavior is apart of the self-concept.

Note: During the course of the phases, the likelihood of people falling back to a previous stage is very real.

Change processes are effective after each stage. I will have to determine the stage at which the person in question is located if I want to change or steer his or her behavior. The likelihood of frequent recurs on is a real but very logical fact. Continue to support and is the message.

Staying alert to pitfalls is the message. It should not be assumed that the inhabitants are very motivated to change. If they're not motivated, they should be given their personal situation. Therefore, workers use interventions that apply to the stage of active change. It is also important to recognize that a person can be at different stages of change, with different problems. It is therefore very important that one can assess the stage at which the person is at.

4.2 THE INTEGRATED MODEL FOR PROMOTING HEALTHY EATING

In order to influence the lifestyle of the participants, I have to focus on the attitude, social skills and own effectiveness of the individual.

Our behavior is affected at both the macro level and[9] the micro level.[10].

For example, if a resident does not have the equipment to prepare a meal or if there are other barriers in the environment, this may prevent a behavioral intent from being converted into behavior.

For example, when one is in the action phase (Figure 2), it is important to improve one's sailing and remove the barrier in order to maintain the existing behavior.

---

[9] At the level of society such as agriculture, economy, trade, policy, etc.
[10] At the level of the individual

This model (De Vries, Dijkstra, & Kuhlman, 1988) also pays attention to individual characteristics. On the basis of this I can check the influence of the knowledge of the resident in quince. Through this way one can see how this person will be influenced by his environment and how he or she assesses himself or herself to change his or her behavior.

A negative in this model is the limited space for the

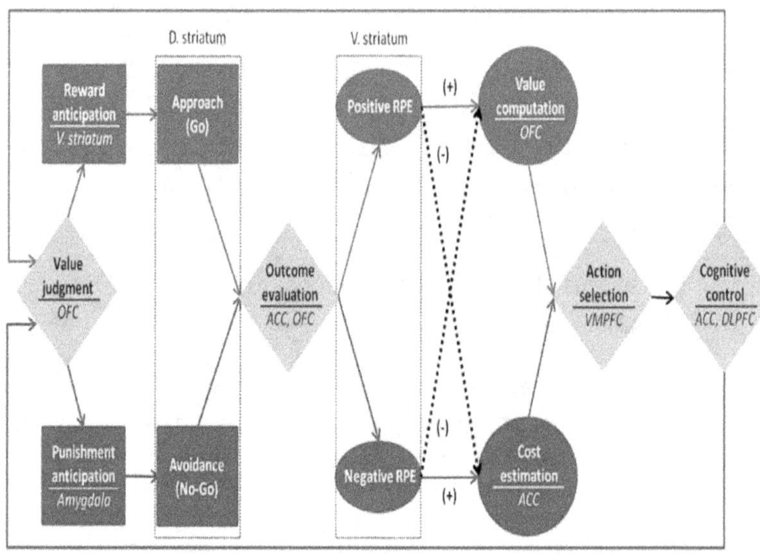

emotional factors that influence the behavior.

FIGURE 2 - Determinant scheme of influences on our behavior

4.2.1 LEGISLATIVE POLICY

When companies or department stores advertise, they must comply with the rules on misleading advertising and comparative advertising. An advertisement is misleading if it makes claims that are incorrect or incomplete.

The supervisory body is here Jep [11].

4.2.2 ECONOMIC INFLUENCES

The economic crisis does not immediately change the purchasing behavior of healthy food. People buy fewer exotic products, the price of which seems to have increased a bit.
Health is the last thing to save. 80% do not go to the doctor any less quickly and the same number of people do not postpone their dental visit. The majority feel that their spending on doctor visits is unchanged from before the economic crisis.

4.2.3 PHYSICAL AVAILABILITY OF FOODSTUFFS

---

[11] The **J**ury for **E**thische **P**advertising is the self-conccipadvertising sector in Belgium. It was founded in 1974 . Advertising Council, which represents the representative associations of the Advertising Council, which represents the representative associations of the

Advertisers, advertising agencies and media group for the purpose of advertising, as a factor of economic and economicto promote ocial expansion. (Jep, 2014)

The food offer but also the price can vary from store to store. Many people will start comparing products in the different supermarkets nearby.

The time aspect is also important.

The time one must do shopping can determine the products one purchases. The way food is depicted in advertising can often be misleading and/or enticing. Some offers are incredibly attractive and advantageous. In this way, one can fall prey to impulse purchases that end up partly in the bin or which are simply unhealthy. Commercial product packaging often places all kinds of claims and logos. They may have different meanings.

Our buying behavior is consciously or unconsciously influenced by this. These things are also all among the influences of physical accessibility of food.

4.2.4 ATTITUDE

Everyone will have their own argument and reason to behave in a certain way. To influence the attitude of a resident, I will have to provide very clear information on the size of the person in question.

By providing this information, the participant will think about his or her own feeding pattern.

4.2.5 SOCIAL INFLUENCE

This component can be subdivided into the social standard, social support by modelling or the exemplary function and by direct social support.

From the perception of the behavior of others and of the norm that prevails in the social group, there will be an influence on one's own behavior.

If I want to change the lifestyle, I will have to find out what the reactions are of his or her immediate environment.

With residents living in a community housing and participating in this project, there will undoubtedly be mutual influence, positive or not.

4.2.6 OWN EFFECTIVENESS

Own effectiveness can best be described as the assessment of how you conduct and/or sustain behavior and how social pressure is resisted.

The participating residents will be more motivated for a act if they feel that they have the ability and skills to carry it out successfully.

This assessment of one's own competence is influenced by observations of others, past experiences, ich amicable sensations and one's own attribution style.

The own attribution style is the way in which one tries to explain one's own behavior from a cause. This can be attributed to itself (internally) or to the environment (externally) (Psychology veer practice, 2004).

These attribution processes play an incredible role in interpreting the client's behavior. As an aid worker one must be aware of one's own attribution processes as well as of the attribution processes of the client.

Of course, I cannot change the behavior of the participating residents from today to tomorrow.

There is a dynamic process in which six different phases are going through.

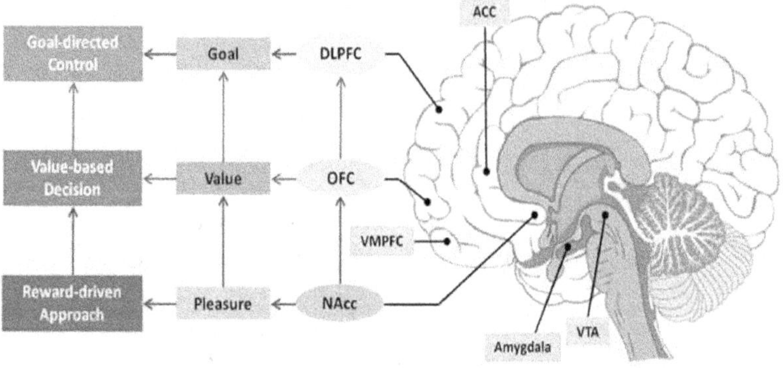

5.1 USE OF ALGORITHMS

The use of an algorithm is essential in determining the stage of behavior change a candidate is at.

In this way, the behavior to be influenced can be responded to more efficiently and effectively.

It is a challenge to find in the dietary behavior a clear standard that can determine what stage a person is in.

With an algorithm I will focus on a certain part of nutrition. This could be fruit or vegetables, for example.

In determining this phase, I will have to question the resident.

So, there will be a subjective assessment (of the resident in question) of the own consumptive as well as a measurement of objective nutrition.

I will apply these algorithms to all parts of the active feed triangle if necessary. The active feeding triangle will be the common thread in determining the correct amounts of nutrients. The active food triangle will be discussed later.

First, I would like to give an example about determining the phase of behavioral change using an algorithm.

For a person between the ages of 19 and 59, the food triangle prescribes 2 to 3 pieces of fruit per day.

I use this algorithm as a guide to interview the resident in
question.

<table>
<tr><td>Question 1: How long have you been eating 2 to 3 pieces of fruit a day?</td></tr>
</table>

√ Yes, Less than 5 months: Action phase

Yes, 6 to 11 months: Phase of conservation

No, or I have no idea Go to question 2

<table>
<tr><td>Question 2: Have you tried to eat more fruit during the last 6 months?</td></tr>
</table>

√ Yes, successfully: Planning phase

√ Yes, without success: Go to question 4

√ No: Go to question 3

<table>
<tr><td>Question 3: Are you thinking of eating more fruit within 6 months?</td></tr>
</table>

❖ Yes:
 Phase of considering
❖ No: Go to question 5

Question 4: Do you really plan to eat more fruit within a period of 6 months?

❖ Yes:
    Planning phase

❖ No: Phase of
    considering

Question 5: Do you think your current intake of fruit is enough?

❖ Yes:
    Phase of preview - unconscious

❖ No;   Phase of fore
    consider – conscious

5.2 TAILORING

Many people are wrongly convinced that they eat healthily and exercise enough. Tailoring uses awareness tests to give [12]these people a clearer picture of their own eating and/or exercise patterns.

These awareness-raising tests are a simple yet indispensable fact in this project. It is a tool in giving the first advice. To change the behavior of

---

[12] In additional Guide you will find these tests.

the people in the long term, it is of course particularly important that after these tests they can count on someone to guide them through the change process.

Different types of tests have been developed.

For example, for all layers of the active food triangle awareness-raising tests (Health Tests, 2011) exist so that one can check to what extent there are shortages for each component.

It is mainly with these tests that I will proceed to determine what phase the participants are in.

This is carried out just before the information session takes place on the subject in question. *For example: When the information session is about fats and fiber, the tests will take place the day before at an individual time.* These tests also serve as a starting point for conversation.

5.3 THE ACTIVE FEEDING TRIANGLE[13]

5.3.1 A DEFINITION

The information model 'The active food triangle' visually gives an idea of what you should eat daily to get enough nutrients and what you need to move daily. (Flemish

---

[13] In additional Guide you will find an overview of the active food triangle.

Institute of Health, 2011)

It is the Supreme Health Council[14] that has drawn up this active food triangle.

It consists of 9 different parts. 8 components relate to food and 1 component relates to physical activity.

The Active Food Triangle is without a doubt the most well-known and most promoted working tool for health promotion.

This model is easy to use for the helper and an accessible medium for the aid worker to reach the rescuer.

Abroad, many other forms have been used: from a circle or a board to a staircase. I am convinced that each of these instruments has its flaws.

---

[14] In Belgium, the High Health Council (HGR) is the scientific advisory body of the Fps Public Health, Safety of the Food Chain and the Environment.

It is not self-evident to put together a model that is scientifically correct and nuanced and at the same time easy to understand.

For myself I see 1 lack in the active feeding triangle. Namely, the emphasis on the use of saturated fats and trans fats.

That is why I discussed it at length at the info sessions.

For the presentation of the information sessions, I call on a handbook recently [15] compiled by approved dieticians.

5.3.3 The active power triangle opposite the power hourglass

The active feeding triangle has been modified 3 times in the last 15 years.

As the research on nutrition is a highly active sector, some things will most likely change.

Two years ago, for example, there was a lot of fuss around the new food hourglass.

Both models offer interesting advantages and disadvantages.

---

[15] Conscious eating – Choose, buy and prepare. First edition was in 2012.

For the residents of sheltered living I have chosen the easiest model to understand and the model that most leans on their budget.

For example, the 'zandloper' model expects the cereal products and potatoes to be avoided while these are cheap products that our residents consume every day. They are asked to replace them with extra vegetables, mushrooms, legumes, tofu or Quorn. The dairy products of the active food triangle should also be replaced by soy products. This would be yet another attack on the limited budget of our candidates. The products of the hourglass model are, in other words, not very accessible to the participants.

So, in addition to the visual advantage, the recommended products in the active food triangle also lean best to this use.

In my view, the food hourglass is of a different level to be included in this Guide and case study as it is designed from a biogerontological [16]point of view.

During this course, graduated in Orthopedagogy, we discussed extensively the active nutrition triangle in semester 3.

----

[16] The study that examines how you can slow down the aging process through sensible eating.

6.1 INFORM AND RAISE AWARENESS

If one wants to change the attitude one must know the active food triangle as well as the principles of balanced nutrition.

I realize this by organizing very accessible information sessions, for up to 3 motivated people, in which different themes are discussed.

This will be 6 information sessions over a period of 6 weeks where different themes will be discussed.

There will be 5 different themes at 5 different times. A general replay will take place at the sixth meeting.

These meetings will take up to an hour and a half and will continue in a meeting room on the institution's domain.

In the ASE model this can be placed under attitude, the knowledge about own eating and exercise behavior.

In the playbook that comes with this thesis, you will find a schematic overview of the necessities for each session.

Each session starts with a foreword and a brief inleading about what we will all deal with.

During these lessons, a presentation will be given at the level of the candidates. These can of course also be found in the playbook that goes with this thesis.

To stay within my mandate of graduated in orthopedagogy, I rely on literature published by a centre of expertise of the Flemish government to compose the presentations. This is partly because we have not had the training to know everything about food. This center of expertise provides information to employees and care workers so that they can in turn give this to the clients.

In this way, the correct information is provided without the need for additional training.

6.1.1 SESSION 1: THE ACTIVE FEEDING TRIANGLE

At the beginning of the lesson, all attendees receive a copy of the active food triangle. When discussing the different groups, we always look at what is in each group, why we need these foods, what to look for and how much we need from each group every day. This copy is then hung in the candidate's personal room (in the room or studio). Later the objectives will be placed next to this which I will write together with the resident. At the end of the lesson, the participants are given a food triangle[17] whose courses have not been filled in and a list of the parts to be filled in.

Together we solve this to see what one has remembered from the lesson.

---

[17] Please consult the playbook for a visual representation.

We will use the active food triangle at every information session and individual moment.

Agenda items: Overview and explanation about the Health Group, Short introduction: The health of the average Belgian, The active nutrition triangle: the phase briefly

____

explained, Pause, Game: Completing the active food triangle, Quiz: Correct or error questions.

Essentials: presentation via PowerPoint, meeting room, projector, laptop, documentation

6.1.2 SESSION 2: EXERCISE AND FLUID

Here, the importance of exercise is shown in combination with daily adequate fluid absorption.

I will ask the candidates what efforts they have made today. They are given time to write this down. We discuss this in groups.

Through PowerPoint I give an overview of light to heavy physical exertion.

During this session we will add up the number of minutes of effort and consider what they might change to their daily lives to have more exercise.

The pros and cons of exercise are displayed through presentation. To

conclude, I let the participants list
some sports they like.

Agenda items: Setting appointments for individual
moments, How does the average Belgian move? The
balance between energy intake and energy absorption,
Movement and absorption of moisture,

Pause, Movie: 10 tips for healthy eating, Quiz with
correct /wrong questions *Essentials*: presentation via
PowerPoint, meeting room, projector, laptop,
documentation.

6.1.3 SESSION 3: FRUIT AND VEGETABLES

During session three we will discuss the importance of
fruits and vegetables. Here, the candidates will have to
take both the fruit and vegetable tests.

The seasons when certain fruits and vegetables are best
purchased are discussed here. Together we will weigh
vegetables with the candidates based on a scale.
Candidates may guess in advance how much a piece of
vegetable will weigh.

Based on a presentation we go over different types of
fruits and vegetables and it their function's.

Agenda items: Discussion of vegetables in the Active food
triangle, Discussion of fruit in the Active Food Triangle,

Discussion of vitamins, minerals, and trace elements,
Pause, Video:
Vitamins, Quiz with correct /wrong questions
Essentials: presentation via PowerPoint, meeting room,
projector, laptop, documentation

6.1.4 SESSION 4: FATS AND FIBER

Here we think about the fats and the fiber. At the
beginning of the lesson, each participant receives the
fiber test. We will fill these out together so that everyone
can see the amount of dietary fiber they take.

Afterwards, I show a few tables that show products with
both low and high dietary fiber.

I will leave the candidates' turn to tell them which one
they think is the best products. I will note this to be used
later in the preparation of the objectives.

We also stop with the fats. We will take a test, just like
the fibers.

Everyone gets the time for this. We will discuss the
results together.

Presentation shows a few tables that show high and low-
fat percentages for different products.

We will discuss all of these and see who
eats how much of what. Here, too, I note
the most important details.

Agenda items: Short Introduction, Where do we find fibers and what do they serve? What does fat and what does it do?, Pause, Movie: Fibers, Quiz with correct / wrong questions

Essentials: presentation via PowerPoint, meeting room, beamer, laptop, documentation

6.1.5 SESSION 5: READING LABELS AND VISITING THE SUPERMARKET

For this session I will collect many different labels from different products. After my explanation about labels and the influence of manufacturers through this label I show the candidates all labels.

They are given time to look at everything to discuss afterwards in group.

The Nutritional Labeling Scheme is also discussed here.

Here, the candidates learn to read the amount of energy displayed per serving as well as the recommended daily amount.

Agenda items: Short introduction, The required data on thelabel, How do you read the nutritional value on the label?, Sample packaging, Best before date, Break, 3 exercises on snacks compare, Video: Read label: Label

Essentials: presentation via PowerPoint, meeting room, projector, laptop, documentation

6.1.6 Session 6: Repetition of the most important data from the previous sessions

What the most important data are will be determined later. This fact depends on the group, were this one had the hardest with it.

I will also let the group decide for themselves which things they would like to have another explanation.

Agenda items: Movement, Water, Cereal products / high fiber products /potatoes, Fruits and vegetables, Dairy products / Meat, fish and meat substitutes, Butter and grease, The residual group, Pause, Movie: Test your common sense 1, Video: Test your common sense 2

Essentials: presentation via PowerPoint, meeting room, projector, laptop, documentation

6.2 PROMOTING EATING AND EXERCISE BEHAVIOR[18]

6.2.1 INDIVIDUAL CONTACT MOMENTS

---

[18] See Annex 2 for a schematic overview of the stages of behavior change and the intervention possibilities of the guidance.

Here, the new insights of one's own eating and exercise behavior are used to deliver bi jdrage to change to a balanced diet and sufficient exercise. The information they receive during the information sessions is thus applicable in daily life and therefore also within the form of sheltered living.

Op the individual contact moments we will examine together and decide on which skills can be worked on.

For example, we will make a shop visit to discover new products.

Organizing cooking moments: learning to prepare new dishes that are delicious, simple, and healthy.

The stages of behavioral change are discussed here to assess the participant's situation.

7.1 THE HEALTH GROUP STARTS

7.1.1 PREPARATION OF INFORMATION SESSIONS

Before I started working out the first goal with great enthusiasm, our team was informed extensively at the team meeting.

Here I explained the Guide , timetable, and objectives of this thesis. The psychological stability of the three candidates as well as their behavior in a group activity were also considered. This is to anticipate anyone listen during the information sessions.

Everything was evaluated positively and my enthusiasm for the project was transferred to the other team members. Expectations are high.

Also, during the first course of semester 8, the start of these information sessions was discussed extensively with my practical supervisors.

This phase of the thesis consists of 6 different information sessions. The three participants were personally invited by me and received an invitation letter with all the information before the start of these information sessions.

All data, documents and tools collected to prepare and prepare the information sessions and individual moments are materials that are scientifically supported by a center of expertise for health promotion and disease prevention of the Flemish government.

In preparation, all useful information is collected from the already indicated reading material and aggregated into a presentation.

Given my limited experience in putting together such a presentation, this preparation phase was already a learning process.

An information session of 1 hour took about 6 hours to gather all the information and necessary material.

These slides are composed in such a way that there is enough explanation to read on it but not too much. It was especially important to take into account the differences in intelligence of the participants.
There is a pretty big difference in level of intelligence associated with cognitive Ability. I tried to stop as much variation as possible in the info sessions with a theoretical part, before the break, and an interactive, more relaxing part after the break. For the interactive part there was footage, games, and quizzes.

Since the total of these presentations involve many pages, they are merged into a separate attachments bundle, the Guide (Objective D), along with the checklist (necessities and steps to be taken for each session) and agenda points.

The day before the information sessions, an individual moment was provided. The intention was to prepare the next session and repeat the previous session briefly. *As an illustration: When the next session will be about fat and and fiber, we do the fat and fiber test together. In this way, the participant knows where he stands compared to the stated standard of the Active Feeding Triangle.*
This is an advantage to discuss the fats and fats in detail a few days later in the group session.
In this way we take the first steps to awareness of your own eating and exercise behavior.

A few days before the information session takes place, I reserve the meeting room where we will start working.

During information sessions I want to organize a cozy atmosphere where hot drinks and water are provided.

Session 1— The active food triangle had calendar items:

-   Overview and explanation about the Health Group
-   Short introduction: The health of the average Belgian
-   The active feeding triangle: the phases briefly explained

- Break
- Game: Completing the active feeding triangle
- Quiz: Right or error questions

During the first group session I will give an explanation about this Guide and case study. Here I inform the participants why the health group has arrived and what the objectives of this thesis are.

At individual moments I had already given an explanation about this project, but it was important to make this even more transparent.

Here the benefits of healthy and balanced diets in the short and long term on human life were listed.

During the sessions I was told that changing some things is not obvious. My job here was to emphasize that 'relapse' or 'relapse' is not a failure but that one can learn from it because it is a normal phenomenon.
I gave examples of re-fall experiences from my own life to show that it occurs in everyone.

It was palpable that the participants looked up to me as a role model for living up to the principles of healthy eating.

That's why I thought it was important to also designer my own process of trial and error to prove just that which is important: learning from oneself in the event of a re-enclosing and not seeing it as an end point.

This allowed me to create a group climate where there was room for understanding and individuality.

When the different phases of the Active feeding triangle were overrun, it was noticeable that it was a long time to listen. There was a lot of information to process during the first 30 minutes, making it difficult to stay attentive.

In preparing this presentation, I had taken this opportunity into account. Therefore, the post-break section was an interactive repetition of the theory.

After the break we started filling in the blank active food triangle using picture cards.

There was a slight panic to be felt at Caroline and Marieke.

It was important here to indicate that it is about getting acquainted with the active nutrition triangle and not a test.

The contrast in cognitive functioning between the candidates was clearly visible. Anneke did the exercise almost perfectly within a short time.

During the first session I occasionally brought tips and tidbits the participants. Reading from the positive reaction of the participants I realized that it would be better to incorporate these into the presentation from the second session onwards. The facts and tips are then processed as their own recognizable colorful slides

between other slides. This creates even more variety in
the presentation.

Session 2 Absorb movement and moisture Calendar:

- Record appointments for individual moments
- How does the average Belgian move?
- The balance between energytake and energy -Recording
- Movement and absorption of moisture
- Break
- Video: 10 tips for healthy eating
- Quiz with correct/for questions

The second session is quite smooth and there is a
lot of interaction among the participants. We
consider the balance that must be present
between the energetic value of the food that one
absorbs and the amount of energy that our body
needs.
I thought it was important to emphasize the absorption
of moisture during this session.

All three participants took the fluid test the day before
the session.

Anneke was ridiculously hard shot from the huge
amounts of coffee she drinks daily.

She seems very convinced she wants to change this.

For myself, this information session was great success. It was clear to see and hear from the participants that this was a huge enrichment.

Session 3 Fruit and vegetablesCalendar:

- Discussion of greens and in the Active Food Triangle
- Discussion of fruit in the Active nutrition triangle
- Discussion of vitamins, minerals and trace elements
- Break
- Video: Vitamins
- Quiz with just / error questions

In preparation for the 3[the] session I had arranged for several vegetable snacks. Cherry tomatoes, carrots, cucumber, radishes, and cauliflower were beautifully presented upon arrival of the participants.

Unfortunately, Marieke was not present at this information session. She was taken to the Psychiatric Center.

Caroline and Anneke were on time and there was enjoyed the treat.

I was hoping to convince them in this way that they are not looking far to find healthy snacks and that they do not have to be expensive.

While discussing the requirements of the active food triangle for the daily absorption of enough vegetables, I use a kitchen scale already to visualize the weight.

I will let everyone guess how many pieces of cauliflower it will take to get to the 300g.

This was an easy exercise for the participants.

I got the most reaction from them when mentioning that the color of fruits and vegetables determines the vitamins that it has.

This allowed them to understand is important to vary in the diet and that it is therefore also 1 of the 3 basic principles of the active dietary triangle.

The video after the break gave a summary of the theory.

The functions of the different vitamins were listened carefully. Of course, it is difficult to remember these things.

That's why I gave the participants and lice cream with the vitamins, their functions and what can cause a deficiency of these vitamins. However, I doubt that it will be used by them later.

Session 4 Fats and fibre - Calendar:

- Letter Introduction
- Where do we find fibres and what are they for?
- What belongs to fat and what does it do?
- Break
- Video: Fibres
- Quiz with correct /wrong questions

The fourth session starts very slowly.

Marieke is still absent due to a hospitalization in the Psychiatric Centre, Anneke was late and Caroline had fallen asleep after her lunch.

After a short telephone contact she arrived during the break. She was very drowsy and slowed down in her reactive and speaking. This is a phenomenon that we see more often with Caroline when she has just woken up.

For her cooperation during this session was difficult. She answered questions briefly and superficially.

The subject of fats and fiber was a lost cause for her to follow. However, she has shown her willingness and motivation to be present.

This was not an obvious and therefore a show of respect.

I try to make the best of it so that Anneke still gets the needed information.

The quiz I only played with her since there came from
Caroline little or no reaction.

When Anneke and Caroline left, I was left with a bad
feeling.

All the hours of preparation for this session suddenly
seemed to me to have been very useless. After a
moment of ventilation with a colleague I came to the
realization that eventually one person understands the
information and has obtained it. The preparation would
have been worth it anyway.

Everyone is present in time and Marieke is also back
from the party. A lot of attention goes to her.

Session 5 label read and visit the supermarket:

- Letter Introduction
- The mandatory dates on the label
- How to you have the nutritional value on the label?
- Sample packaging
- The best-before date
- Break
- 3compare exercises on snacks
- Movie: Read label

Caroline and Anneke show their concern and are happy
to be back.

Marieke stays up for the entire hour and often asks when the break starts. She is constantly distracted and talks about various topics that do not relate at all to the health group.

The tears often jump into her eyes without a specific reason.

I do not immediately follow up on this in the hope that my explanation and the presentation will distract her thoughts.

The downside to this session, however, is that itis a long piece of theory before the break. This one is the longest of them all.

That is why I've been going over some pieces a bit faster and I've expanded the most important things a bit.

Like the piece on the light products.

It was important to explain the common misunderstandings and errors surrounding the use of light products.

Session 6- Repetition: The Active Feeding Triangle

- Movement
- Water
- Graan products / high fibre products / potatoes
- Fruit and vegetables
- Milk products / Meat, fish and meat substitutes
- Butter and grease
- The remaining
- Break
- Video: Test your common sense 1
- FiMP: Test your common sense 2

The purpose of this session was to give a solid repetition about all the layers of the feeding triangle that we have seen until then.

For Anneke, this repetition was really an unnecessary thing. Also during the individual contact moments, it had become clear that she knows the active feeding triangle very well. This was not noticeable to her during the session and she respected the fact that for the other participants a repetition is welcome.

At the start of the info sessions there was a lot of interest from colleagues. For example, there were numerous informal consultation moments in function of the health group. Informal consultation moments are a quite common and typical phenomenon within our setting of sheltered living.

This is since within this setting the colleagues do not work 'side-by-side', but each offers separate guidance in the homes and/or studios.

This way of working is often common within forms of housing such as sheltered living or outpatient home care.

In addition to these informal consultations, formal consultations have of course also taken place.

The team's relationship with the health group is ensured by 2 of the 4 objectives I have set out.

The realization of this can be found in point 8.2, objectives achieved.

8.1 Result of the health group on the participants and advice for further guidance.

8.1.1 HEALTH GROUP RESULT ON CAROLINE

Caroline lost 9 kg at the start of her participation because of a persistent flu. She is on the verge of full recovery at the start of her participation but no longer has the courage and desire to cook.

The simplicity and comfort that ready meals offer are not in this.

Her diet is very one-sided, but she has already made some attempts to eat more vegetables, for example.

Caroline now tries to leave the bike at home and go to the store on foot. So that she gets closer to 30 minutes of moderate intensity movement per day.

For Caroline, losing weight is often more important than knowing she is healthy.

At Caroline everything must remain very simple, otherwise she quickly loses the courage to do it.

To eat more balanced, she has now switched to frozen vegetables and herself sliced potatoes instead of ready meals.

With Caroline state also a shop visit on the program to discover new products together to create simple and healthy menus.

The combination of her obesity, heavy medication, and mental state costs her an incredible amount of energy.

Despite all this, she indicates that she would like to continue with the health group and does not regret her choice to participate.

Advice for further guidance
At Caroline, the focus will be on providing even further information about wat healthy food is so that she can better see the benefits and not just 'lose weight'. In her guidance it is important to indicate that everything needs time.

The further transfer of knowledge and information about nutrition is necessary when it can become even more detached from its one-sided diet.

Continuing to motivate small changes remains the message here because recurring is a periodic phenomenon.

There is a very motivated Anneke who already knows the active food triangle from the outside and tries to apply as much as possible in everyday life.

She used to drink a lot of coffee all day with little water. This is now reversed where coffee is limited to 2 to 3 bags per day.

She consciously eats 2 pieces of fruit daily and tries to do 30 minutes of moderate exercise. She still takes the bus every day but gets on, at another stop so that she can continue foot. She looses herself in eating sweets or burgers in a very short time with a feeling of guilt as a result.

The daily intake of the drug Olanzapine may play a large role in this.

Fortnightly she will walk for 40 to 50 minutes.

This is the highest possible frequency for her because the physical recovery takes its toll on her psychological stability.

Advice for further guidance
Temporizing the urge to lose weight is the message.

For further individual working, the focus here is on your own effectiveness in the preparation of healthy food.

Organizing a cooking moment can be a great added value for her if the preparation of new, healthy, and simple dishes can be explored here.

At Anneke, the focus will be more on further exploring what she wants to achieve and why as well as continuing to motivate them to keep the current changes.

One has to be alerted all the time because the relapse in binges is always lurking around the corner. This with her negotiable , can provide new possibilities for intervention in the future.

8.1.3 HEALTH GROUP RESULT ON MARIEKE

Marieke did less well psychologically and physically.

During the period of the development of this integrated competency test, she went into hospital.

This admission is separate from her participation in the health group.

Due to her absence and decompensation, Marieke could not be trusted with the active food triangle. As a result, she has taken some of the information with her and does not know what she wants and can achieve with it.

In this way, we can hopefully shift the focus to the benefits of certain eating or exercise behavior to start again.

However, the information sessions and our individual contact moments were an added value in function of her gradual return from the psychiatric center to her studio.

Advice for further guidance

Re-listening to her positive and negative arguments can serve as a starting point for a new start.

A new participation in the health group has been designated to ensure meaningful daycare as the lapse in loneliness id and depression is a real danger. In this way she gets a new opportunity to get to know the active food triangle better.

√ Objective A: To inform and sensitize the participants of the project has been achieved.

All sessions have taken place with the necessary attendees. Since there is a promotion of eating– and exercise behavior, the prior informing and sensitizing has thus proven its usefulness.

The presence and cooperation of the participants:

- ➤ Anneke participated in all 6 information sessions.
- ➤ Caroline missed 1/2 information session.
- ➤ Marieke missed 2 information sessions.

- ❖ Goal B: To promote eating and exercise behavior has been achieved.

The goal has been achieved in the short and medium term. To speak of the preservation (long-term objective) of these behavioral changes, an evaluation is needed after a period of 6 months.

During the period of the information sessions, changes in the eating and exercise behavior of the participants were already visible.

These changes were present earlier in the timetable of this thesis than planned at this point I had not yet approached anyone directly to change things in one's own lifestyle. These first changes were due to the participation in the health group. In point 8.4 you will find an additional comment on this objective.

- ❖ Goal C: To include changes and objectives in the client's guidance plan has been achieved.

To guarantee the continuity of the objectives and to maintain the change process of the participants, it is important to include them in the individual guidance plans.

- ❖ Goal D: Drawing up a Guide for the health group has been achieved

You can find the Guide in the attached annex bundle. It includes all the aspects and characteristics that a Guide needs to be fun, namely: an overview of all direct preparatory activities, PowerPoint slides, attachments, nutrition tests as well as an overview of the necessary material for each session, all information about the target group, the health problem and the goal to be achieved.

8.3 UNDISCLOSED OBJECTIVES

Despite very minimal changes in Marieke's eating and exercise behavior, it can be argued that the proposed objective B, promoting eating and exercise behavior, has not been real for her situation.

Her participation in the information sessions and individual moments was too limited to make the most of its benefits.

However, the reason for her limited participation was beyond the influence of the health group to respond to this.

8.4 PROCESS EVALUATION

The use of algorithms is quite a static fact. Here, closed
questions are asked, so that the dialogue is not. It is a
very direct and confrontational way to check the eating
behavior. These algorithms would not be a good means
of use in people who do not know or are only limited.
These may give a false impression because one may
come across as a supervisor.
I did not feel that any of the participants, through this
Guide and case study, felt judged.

Of course, after taking these tests, we were able to start
a conversation about the subject of the test.

This made it possible to dwell on the subject for a longer
time

The stages of behavior change were an interesting
means of theoretically approaching the participant's
situation.

Because I have a coaching style with which I
come across very naturally with the participants,
this creates a space in which there is quick trust
and confidence. This model made the most sense
to find out what stage the person is in. The
recommended approach to moving to the next
phase was useful to keep in mind at all but the
targeted approach came rather spontaneously.

Aim C, changes and objectives included in the client's guidance plan and goal D, drawing up a Guide for the health group, have been drawn up with a view to the future. At goal C, several colleagues are reached. Here, the colleagues who have been made responsible for the annual renewal and adaptation of a resident's guidance plan. These are the people who meet them the most. This idea was proposed and unanimously approved at a team meeting.

In this way, the objectives and changes are continued and assured by this being an annual fact in which follow-up is provided for in the individual guidance.

If my employment stops by sheltered living, the achievement of Objective D ensures that the health group makes its way through a colleague. She has been appointed at her own request.

In this way, the choice was made quickly because they have a great personal interest nutrition and diet.

We have a mutual agreement to guarantee the transfer of the Guide and additional explanation.

All information can be found digitally on the server of sheltered living so that one has the possibility to adjust.

All information refers to the entire package. This is about personal observations, presentations, attachments, and documents needed for the correct and responsible development of the health group.

Because both companies provide a sustainable and permanent method for further follow-up, I am convinced that within 1 year the health group will not be a bygone initiative but an established value within sheltered living.

With the start-up of the health group I wanted to set out a Guide that is needed for my further successor.

This is intended as a guide to continue this project.

Sheltered Housing is a form of housing in which the inhabitants experience a lot of freedom and independence.

This way of working is palpable in this thesis in the sense that one must be able to let go of the process of change to a certain extent.

One only encounters the participants 2 to 3 times a week. Despite these contact moments, which last up to an hour and a half, this turns out to be enough to follow the process of change.
The residents experience a feeling of control.

Observations in this project teach me that the participation in the information sessions meant a greater added value than first thought. The participants experience social support here which benefits from their own motivation to continue.

For such a project I would have liked to work even more intensively individually to achieve even more results.

There is a lot of responsibility on the part of the resident which can be a pitfall for the guidance. One must remain attentive so that the guidance does not take over too much from the resident, so that he can take the necessary steps in the process himself.

I hope that the realization and my work can contribute to the quality, stability, and wellbeing of life for the clients.

Literature list

Retrieved from Jep: http://www.jep.be/nl/

Picked up from pharmacotherapeutic compass:
        https://www.farmacotherapeutischkompas.nl/inleidend
        eteksten/i/inl%20anxiolytica.asp

(2004). In J. Rigter, *Psychology for practice* (pp. 170 - 171).
Amsterdam: Coutinho e.g.

(2012). In S. Claes, E. Constant, P. Cosyns, A. De Nayer, M.
        Dierick, & D. Souery, *Manual psychopharmacology* (pp.
        153 - 179). Ghent: Academia press.

Bayingana, K., Demarest, S., & Gisle, L. (2004). *Health survey
through an interview.* Brussels: Scientific

        Institute for Public Health. 10, 2014,from http://zorg-en-
        gezondheid.be/cijfers.aspx

Beers, M., Jones, T., & Berkwits, M. (2008). *Inform health care
        providers about the recommendations for nutrition and
        exercise.* Retrieved from http://www.zorg-

        engezondheid.be/uploadedFiles/NLsite_v2/Gezond_leve
        n_en_milieu/Gezonde_voeding_en_ movement/Food
        expert%20project%20consensustext%2025-07-2012.pdf

Boevinck, W., Wolf, J., C, v. N., & A, S. (1995, Feb. *Quality of life
        of long-term outpatient*and dependent*psychiatric
        patients; a conceptual exploration.* Called on 7
        November 2014, from Journal of Psychiatry:
        http://www.tijdschriftvoorpsychiatrie.nl/issues/196/artic
        les/955

Buziarsist, J., & Gisle, L. (2001). *Health survey dear means of Interview*. Brussels: Scientific Institute of Public Health.

Cahn, W., Ramlal, D., Bruggeman, R., De Haan, I., Scheepers, F. E., & Van Soest, M. M. (2008). Prevention and treatment of somatic complications in antipsychotic use. *Tid for psychiatry*,579 - 591.

De Vries, H., Dijkstra, M., & Kuhlman, P. (1988). Self efficacy: The third factor besides attitudes and subjective norm as a predictor of behavioral intentions. Maastricht: University of Limburg.

European Commision. (2007, 05 30). Summoned on 17 September 2014, from http://ec.europa.eu/health/ph_determinants/life_style/nutrition/keydocs_nutrition_en.ht m *Health tests*. (2011). Summoned on October 5, 2014, from http://gezondheidstest.be/tests_alle.html

(2014).). *Annual report*.

Prochaska, J., Norcross, J., & Diclemente, C. (1994). Picked up from Healing unleashed: http://healingunleashed.com/wp-content/uploads/2014/03/CHANGE-BOOK.pdf

Psychiatric function disorders in vulnerable elderly people. (2010). In T. Bakker, H. Diesfeldt, & D. Sipsma. Axes: Van Gorcum.

Van Der Veen, M., & Goijarts, F. (2008). Motivational conversation for social agogic work. Bohn Stafleu from Loghum. Retrieved from http://www.skillscascade.com/handouts/StagesofChangeModel.htm

Vdab. (2010). Retrieved from
https://www.vdab.be/sites/web/files/doc/trends/KiK_La
aggeschoolden201002.pdf

*Flemish Institute of*Health. (2011). Summoned on 17 October
2014, from
http://www.vigez.be/voeding_en_beweging/actieve_vo
edingsdriehoek

Appendix 1: Usual antipsychotic medication and their effects

Generic name Productname	Weight steam E	Lipid - The Future	Risk Diabetes	Eps
Aripiprazol Abilify	/ ?	0 / ?	?	+ / -
Broomperido	+ / -	0	?	+++
Clozapin	+++	++	++	0
Flufenazine Anatensol	+	+ / -	?	++
Haloperidol Haldol	+ / -	0	+ / -	+++
Levomepromazi E	++	++	++	++
Olanzapine Zyprexa	+++	++	++	+ /
Perfenazine	+ / -	0	+ / -	++
Pimozide Orap	0	0	+ / -	+++
Risperiddor Risperdal	++	+ / -	+ / -	++
Sertindo	+	?	?	0
Quetiapine Seroquel	++	+	+	0
Sulpiride	+ / -	0	?	+ / -
Zuclopentixol Clopixol	+ / -	0	?	+++

Phase of Behavior Change	Interventions at each transition	What I MUST do	What I'm NOT allowed to do
Preview GOAL: think about the problem. What and why you want to change a certain behavior	Informing, sensitizing and accepting E.g. The information sessions	Giving personal information and use of the Awareness. (see Tailoring chapter). Here I give the person the space to express his feelings to express about unwanted behavior and the need to Change. I can't force anyone to resist here.	I can't assume that the person in question has all the knowledge about a healthy lifestyle. The feelings and emotional I certainly cannot ignore justification.

| **Consider**
GOAL: decide to start with small changes | Here I will have to detect the barriers and barriers.

This allows me to increase confidence in my own ability to

effectively implement changes. | Highlight the benefits to balanced eating: influence on the health and fitness. Discuss the barriers and solve it together. Giving positive Feedback. Motivating social support.

Clarifying contradictions and opposites

about the desired behavior and the | I can't underestimate the impact of the environment. People living in a community house live will be faced daily and be seduced by the eating behavior of the inmates.

I should not worry about the person's conflicting ideas. |
| | | emphasize benefits. | |

Plans PURPOSE: The behavior to change is scheduled for execution	Here I will see the conflicting ideas try to avoid and draw up an action plan.	The resident may have his own concrete and feasible set objectives. Importantly here, I have small rewards changes. Every change is a step Forward. Further stimulating the person and support in this change.	Don't ask for vague behavioral changes. For example, "Eat more vegetables." Any change is good, so never say it's not good enough.

Acting / Action TARGET: behavior prevent relapse	Learning skills and expanding social support	Refer to educational programs. Self-help materials. The resident would to show interest in leaflets, etc. Learning to deal with temptations. Learn skills.	Don't just give the person information.
Maintain GOAL: long-term behavior retention, preventing relapse	Learning problem-solving skills and building social and environmental support.	Teach the person to anticipate and assess risk situations. Encourage the person to regroup in the event of a reattack.	First action does not equal lasting change.